Low Carb Diet Guide:
The Ultimate 7 Day Guide to Jump-Start Fat Loss Fast and Start Feeling Great Today

Henry Brooke

Table of Contents

Table of Contents

Introduction

Chapter 1: How Low Carb Diets Help With Weight Loss

Chapter 2: Choosing the Low Carb Options for Meal Time

    Going to the Grocery Store

    Cleaning Out Pantry

    One Week Meal Plan

Chapter 3: Adding more Activity to Get Greater Results

Chapter 4: Easy Recipes to Get Started

    Breakfasts

    Lunch

    Dinner

    Dessert

Conclusion

Introduction

Many of the diet plans out there are wrong. You have been told for years that eating plenty of carbs and cutting out the fat is the best and only way to lose weight. Unfortunately, many of you fall for this and are disappointed when you are not losing the weight that you want. There is a solution though. The low carb diet is an alternative that you can trust and turn to when other diet plans have failed you. It goes off the opposite idea; instead of carbs being good and fats being bad, the low carb diet sees carbs as the problem and asks you to reduce them down. This guidebook will provide you more information on this great diet plan and how it can help you to lose the weight that you want.

In this guidebook, you will find all of the information that you need about the low carb diet and how it can benefit you. First, you will learn what the low carb diet is and how it can help you to lose weight. Once you are hooked, it provides some help on how to go grocery shopping, empty out your pantry, and a sample menu plan for a week so you can get started. Also, don't forget the information in chapter 3 that helps you to realize that you still need to get up and get moving for weight loss even with this amazing diet plan. Finally, there are 20 delicious recipes at the end for breakfast, lunch, dinner, and of course dessert, so you can really get going on the right track with this plan.

Use this guidebook today to finally lose the weight that you have always wanted without all of the disappointments that come with being on other kinds of weight loss and diet plans.

Chapter 1: How Low Carb Diets Help With Weight Loss

With all of the weight loss diets and products that are on the market, it can be difficult to tell which ones are going to be able to help you and which ones will just add on more of the weight. Each of the diet programs and pills promises to be the best, but some are even harmful to your health. Millions of people buy into these weight loss solutions and often they do not see the results that they are looking for. The solution is simple; you are just eating the wrong kinds of food.

Most people who go on a diet are going to concentrate just on eating fewer fats. They think that fat is the enemy and will cut it out almost completely, without seeing the results that they want. This is because they are starving out the body from the fat that it needs to survive while at the same time increasing the amounts of carbs that are being consumed. The real enemy to your diet is not the fat, it is the carbs that are consumed.

A low carb diet is the perfect solution for losing weight; depending on the specific diet you choose, it is possible to avoid other health concerns such as metabolic syndrome and diabetes as well. There are many reasons why you would want to follow a diet that is low in carbs including:

- You are interested in a diet that will restrict the amounts of carbs you are consuming in order to lose weight.
- You think that changing your old eating habits is important in order to be healthier.
- You like the foods that are offered in a low carb diet and eating fewer carbs makes sense to you in terms of weight loss.

So how does eating fewer carbs help with you staying healthy and losing weight? The issue is not necessarily carbs, it is possible to get plenty of nutrients from the carbs you eat, the issue is that many of the carbs found in food products are simple ones. These are the kinds that are basically just fancy sugars that will slow down your metabolism and add on the weight. Simple carbs are the enemy to your body and eating foods such as sodas, juices, candy, cake, cookies, pasta, and white bread.

Your body will use carbs as a way to fuel itself and keep going. The starches and sugars found in many of the carbs in your body will be broken down so they become sugars in digestion before being absorbed into the bloodstream and turned into glucose. This glucose is going to raise the blood sugar so that insulin is released and the glucose can then going to fuel some of the body cells. If you take in too much, which can easily occur while eating the foods listed above, it is just going to be stored in your muscles and liver until you end up using it, or it can be converted into fat if left there long enough.

The idea with a low carb diet is that you are decreasing the amount of carbs in your diet so that you can lower the levels of insulin. This will cause the body to burn off the stored up fat to get more energy and will lead to weight loss if it is done right. Simple idea in thought, but cutting out those treats and sodas can be difficult at first.

Each of the diets you go on will have different requirements for the carbs that you will need to consume. Some will start out with almost nothing, such as the South Beach and Atkins Diets only allowing a cup of vegetables for the whole day for carbs. Most of these will restrict severely the first few weeks and then you can add more in to the diet as you go. The idea behind these extremes is restricting this much makes it easier to stay in a good level once carbs are allowed back into the diet.

While you are on these low carb diets, you will need to concentrate on other food groups in order to get the nutrients that your body needs. Some good options to stay healthy and full on a low carb diet will include vegetables without a lot of starch, eggs, fish, poultry, and meat. For the most part you will have to cut out your grains, at least in the beginning to comply with the rules of this diet.

Basically, this kind of diet is asking you to change the way that you think about carbs as well as the types of food you are eating. Not all carbs are going to be eliminated (this would be almost impossible and not that healthy considering fruits and vegetables contain carbs in them), but rather to think about the carbs you are consuming and making smart decisions for your overall health.

Choosing complex carbs is the way to go on a low carb diet. Since you are only allowed a certain amount of carbs into the diet, it is important that you make the right decisions. You will not have enough of an allowance on most of these diets to eat a bunch of donuts or consume as much pop as you would like. Instead, you must choose the carbs, such as fruits and vegetables that provide your body with the nutrition it needs and which can also fill you up for much longer than simple carbs.

Why is it so important to choose complex carbs? Unlike the simple carbs which will build up and cause fat to be in the body, and therefore more weight, complex carbs will almost do the opposite and can work well with the ideas of this diet and weight loss. The complex carbs have a lot of fiber, as well as other nutrients. This means that you can eat just a small amount and be full for longer, even though fewer calories are being consumed. This is critical to weight loss and could be the answer you need.

So what foods can I eat on the low carb diet? Am I able to eat as much fat as I want and lose weight? While you are cutting out a major part of a food group from your diet, this does not give you a license to eat whatever you want. It is all about control and moderation as well as staying healthy in order to get the weight loss. While fat is going to be an important ingredient in this diet, it is all about choosing the right kinds of fat and in the right amounts. The diets that fall under this category are not going to allow you to go and get a huge fast food hamburger every night and then you will lose weight. Fat is not the enemy here, but you need to pick the right kinds of fat.

Some good options for eating on this diet is to include lots of fruits and vegetables. These have the nutrients your body needs in a healthy way. Plus they are low on calories but will fill you up so it is easier to lose weight. Options like lean meats, low fat milks and cheeses, seafood, a few nuts each day, and some whole grain and multigrain choices for your carbs can be great additions.

Basically, this diet is going to help you to lose weight because you are cutting out the simple carbs, the ones that build up in the body and cause you to get fat, and instead is asking you to replace with healthy eating options. When the simple carbs are reduced, you will force the body to start burning fat cells and losing weight. It is simple to understand but will take some time to put into practice for weight loss success.

Chapter 2: Choosing the Low Carb Options for Meal Time

While the thoughts behind a low carb diet are easy to understand, it can actually be difficult to make your meals work without carbs. Think about it; how many meals have you done that include some form of rice, pasta, or bread? The answer is probably quite a few so getting the right foods can take some time to get used to. This chapter is going to help you to make the right choices at meal time in order to get the best health and to see the best results on a low carb diet plan.

Going to the Grocery Store

Going to the grocery store is probably going to be the hardest thing for you to do when first starting on a low carb diet. You are probably used to going to certain areas of the store for your food and now you need to be in different areas and will spend a lot of time looking at labels to make sure that no hidden carbs are there. Don't worry, while the first few trips might be a pain to get used to, after a few times you will know what you can have and where it is located and the process will become much easier.

When you are at the grocery store, try to stick near the perimeter. This is the area where the fresh and health products are going to be located. Each grocery store might have a slightly different layout, but all of them will keep the processed and high carb foods in the middle aisles while the outer layers will have the lean meats, fish, vegetables, fruits, milks, yogurts, eggs, and other healthy options. Try to stick to these outside aisles and only go into the first few aisles if you really need to. This is a good and quick way to get the food that you need without having to think about it too much.

Also, before you head out to the store, make a grocery list. Do some surfing on the web or look at the recipes at the end of this guidebook and then pick the ingredients that you need from there. Any recipe that you are using should be low fat so double check on this point; you would hate to ruin all of your hard work by having the wrong recipes. Take this list to the grocery store with you and stick with it. This will make the experience easier plus will ensure that you are getting quality and low carb food.

Cleaning Out Pantry

When starting a low carb diet, you may also want to consider cleaning out the pantry. Looking through the pantry, you may notice that there are a lot of unhealthy foods and snacks inside that would not match up to your new diet plan. Taking the time to get rid of them right away can help avoid temptation later on. It is hard to say no to a treat, especially when you are on a diet, when that treat is right there in your pantry.

The low carb diet is going to ask you to consume a lot of fresh ingredients so you might have to get rid of a lot of the meals that are inside. Be careful and picky and get rid of anything that might throw your plans off track. If you do not feel comfortable throwing out food, consider boxing it up and sending it to the local food bank so others can benefit off what you are not allowed to have. While you are at it, clean out the cupboards, fridge, and freezer as well for the best results.

Sometimes the hardest part about beginning a new diet plan is that you are not sure what you should eat and what you should avoid. While the low carb diet is pretty basic, you still need to come up with some meal options, and cooking without carbs can be a challenge. Here is a weeks' worth of meals, including breakfast, lunch, and dinner to help make the transition to low carb easier.

Monday

Breakfast: a small omelet with mixed vegetables. Fry it in coconut oil or butter.
Lunch—a small salad with vegetables with a side of yogurt and blueberries topped with a small amount of almonds.
Dinner—a cheeseburger, without a bun, topped with a salsa sauce and a few vegetables on the side.

Tuesday

Breakfast—bacon and eggs
Lunch—eat some of the leftovers from the night before, including plenty of vegetables and a few fruits if you would like.
Dinner: fresh salmon with a little butter on top and a side of vegetables.

Wednesday

Breakfast—eggs with lots of vegetables, fried in either coconut oil or butter
Lunch--a big salad with shrimp and a bit of olive oil
Dinner—grilled chicken with some vegetables and a small salad topped with strawberries.

Thursday

Breakfast—omelet with vegetables of your choice, fried in some coconut oil
Lunch—homemade smoothie made with protein powder, almonds, berries, and coconut milk; 1 serving.
Dinner—steak with a little bit of fat and a side of veggies.

Friday:

Breakfast--bacon and eggs of your choice and a few veggies if you would like.
Lunch: yogurt topped with some walnuts, coconut flakes, and berries.
Dinner—meatballs on a bed of vegetables of your choice.

Saturday
Breakfast: omelet with lots of vegetables
Lunch: chicken salad, large, with a bit of vegetable oil for dressing
Dinner—pork chops with some vegetables and fruit

Sunday

Breakfast: Bacon and eggs
Lunch: a homemade smoothie with some coconut milk, berries, protein powder that is chocolate, and some heavy cream
Dinner: chicken wings grilled and a bit of spinach on the side.

As you can see, there are plenty of great meals to enjoy while on a low carb diet. Your meals do not need to be boring in order to meet recommendations, you just have to be smart about what you are serving.

Chapter 3: Adding more Activity to Get Greater Results

In order to really see the weight loss that you want, it is important that you not only eat the right foods, but that you include some form of physical activity into your routine as well. Exercise is so critical whether you are just trying to get healthy or lose weight so adding it into your routine can make so many things better. This chapter will spend some time discussing how to add in more activity to your day for the best health and weight loss results.

When you first get started, you need to be careful about how quickly you are dropping off the carbs when it comes to your energy levels. If you drop below 100 grams of carbs, you will see that the glucose and its stores are going down quickly, which can result in some great weight loss, but you will also see a loss in energy and how well you can work out. This is because the body is getting used to not having its main source of energy and is switching over to using the fat stores in your body. Give it a few days, your energy will not be gone forever and you will see some renewed energy in no time.

What this means for you is you will need to take exercising a little bit slow when you first start out. Your body is going to be worn and tired from the lack of carbs and while it is in this transition period, you will feel lethargic and more likely to get an injury. It is probably best to skip the gym for the first few days on the diet, but if you go, take it slow and just do some gently workouts. Over time you will get your energy back and will be able to work out as hard as you used to.

On a low carb diet, longer and low intensity workouts may be the best bet for you. This is because these kinds of diets are going to take more fat to burn and less carbs. After you have adapted to not having a lot of carbs in your diet, it does not make as much sense to try and get rid of them and instead you will want to burn up the extra fat that you are taking in. Low intensity workouts that last a longer amount of time can do this.

To make sure that you are staying in the right zone, you should keep your heart rate at between 65 and 70 percent of its maximum. This will result in the amount of energy you are using being split up with 40 percent coming from carbs and the other 60 percent coming from the fat. This will help to continue the weight loss that you have started and won't waste up all of the carbs and the carbs nutrition you are taking in.

For some people, it is not a good idea to do a hardcore strength training plan when you are on a low carb diet because the two do not mix that well. Eating fewer carbs seems to lead to a lowering of testosterone levels which can result in muscle loss. This can make it difficult to do the strength training that you need. These exercises are still important to your body so it is important that you do them, but keep safe. When you are planning on doing some strength training, eat the majority of your daily carbs, such as fruits and vegetables, right before you go and workout. Do this about an hour or two before lifting and then do it again about an hour afterwards in order to keep the muscles strong and growing while you do these types of workouts.

Working out is important when you are on any diet and it is just as true on a low carb diet. You just need to be careful when you are first starting out. Your body is not used to eating lower amounts of carbs and it might not be ready for the changes. You might experience less energy and endurance at first, but it will come back once the body adapts to the changes. Take it slow for the first couple of weeks and soon your energy will be back and you can lose weight in no time.

Chapter 4: Easy Recipes to Get Started

Breakfasts

Scrambled Eggs and Hash Browns

Ingredients:

1 Tbsp. onion
1 c. rice
2 eggs
2 Tbsp. butter
Pepper
Salt

Directions:

To begin this recipe, heat up a little bit of butter on a skillet before adding the onion and the rice. Cook these ingredients until both are browned.

At this time, break the eggs into the mixture, making sure to stir in order to scramble up the eggs well.

Cook until the eggs are completely done. Right before serving, season with some pepper and salt and then enjoy!

Avocado Scrambled Eggs

Ingredients:

2 eggs
½ Tbsp. butter
½ avocado
½ red bell pepper
Salt

Directions:

Bring out a skillet and warm up some butter on it. When the butter is melted, break your eggs in the pan, making sure to break up the yolks using a spoon before sprinkling on some salt.

Scramble up the eggs and continue to do this until the eggs begin to set up. At this time you will want to quickly add the avocado and the peppers to the mixture.

Cook all of these ingredients until the eggs are done, taking time to adjust the seasoning to your liking. Serve this right away.

Muenster Omelet

Ingredients:

¼ red pepper
2 sliced diced deli ham
4 cherry tomatoes
2 eggs
2 tsp. chopped yellow onion
Salt
Pepper
2 Tbsp. milk
1 ¼ c. Muenster cheese

Directions:

Begin this recipe by bringing out a skillet and sautéing together the onions, tomatoes, pepper, and ham until they become soft.

In a bowl, mix together the eggs and the milk before adding into the vegetable mixture. Cook both sides of the eggs until well done.

Add the cheese to this mixture and allow it some time to melt before serving.

Hash Brown Cakes

Ingredients:

½ onion
1 lb. red potatoes
1 Tbsp. olive oil
¼ tsp. salt
2 tsp. thyme
1/8 tsp. pepper

Directions:

To begin this recipe, turn on the oven and let it heat up to 300 degrees. While the oven is heating up, peel and shred the potatoes before rinsing off with cold water and placing into the bowl. Stir the pepper, salt, thyme, oil, and quartered onion into the bowl with the potatoes.

Heat up a skillet before scooping a tablespoon of your potatoes mixture onto the surface. Press the mixture down and then allow it to cook for about 5 minutes.

When the one side is done, turn it over and give it time to cook for another 5 minutes so that it becomes golden brown.

Place your potato cakes onto a baking sheet before placing into the oven to bake for about 10 minutes or until done. Serve warm.

Eggplant Parmesan

Ingredients:

Salt
Oil
1 lb. eggplant
Garlic powder
3 oz. mozzarella cheese
6 Tbsp. tomato sauce
2 Tbsp. Parmesan

Directions:

Start this recipe by slicing up the eggplant into thin slices. Salt each side and then place into a coriander for 30 minutes. After this time you can pat the eggplant dry and place onto a baking sheet.

Turn on the oven and let it preheat to 350 degrees. After arranging the eggplant onto the baking sheet and seasoning with the garlic powder, some tomato sauce, and the mozzarella cheese before topping with another piece of eggplant, place the baking sheet into the oven.

Bake the eggplant for around 10 minutes so that the cheese can melt before enjoying.

Thai Salad

Ingredients:

½ c. bean sprouts
1 c. spinach
½ red pepper
4 Tbsp. hot chilies
¾ c. green onions
1 c. carrots
2 c. cabbage, shredded
½ cucumber
Bok choy
Thai Dressing
3 Tbsp. oil
¼ c. lime juice
1 Tbsp. sesame oil
2 tsp. Splenda
1 Tbsp. soy sauce
1 small chili
Ginger
Cilantro

Directions:

Start this recipe by making the dressing. Do this by whisking together the dressing ingredients and setting aside.

Next, bring out another bowl and mix together the vegetables. Toss the dressing in with the vegetables and let it marinate for at least an hour in the refrigerator. Enjoy the salad once it has had time to marinate.

Big Mac Bowl

Ingredients:

Salt
Pepper
½ lb. ground beef
1 slice American cheese
46 grams pickle slices
1 Tbsp. dry onions
1 ½ oz. iceberg lettuce
2 Tbsp. Thousand Island Dressing

Directions:

Start this recipe by browning up the ground beef, taking the time to drain any fat off before seasoning with some pepper and salt.

While the beef is cooking, you can soak the onions in the water in order to rehydrate them. Add the cheese to the meat and let it cook for a few seconds until it begins to melt.

Place the meat into a big bowl and add the rest of the ingredients in with it. Toss everything together and serve right away.

Shrimp Scampi

Ingredients:

¼ tsp. garlic powder
2 Tbsp. butter
Salt
Pepper
Cayenne
½ lb. cooked shrimp
Parsley

Directions:

Bring out a skillet and heat up the butter onside. Add the garlic powder and the shrimp to the skillet and let it cook on a high setting until there is a little bit of sauce left.

After this time, you can reduce the heat and season with the cayenne, pepper, and salt. Sprinkle with the parsley right before serving.

Chicken Enchilada Casserole

Ingredients:

2 tsp. taco seasoning
4 c. cooked chicken
9 oz. cream cheese
7 oz. Green Mexican Salsa
1 Tbsp. chives
6 oz. Monterey Jack cheese
4 oz. green chilies
4 green onions

Directions:

Turn on the oven and let it heat up to 350 degrees. Take out a baking pan and great is up before placing the chicken inside and tossing with some taco seasoning.

Next, soften up the cream cheese before placing into a bowl with the green sauce and the chives, making sure to whisk hem together well. Stir the chilies in next.

Pour this sauce over the chicken and top with some cheese. Bake the dish for 25 minutes so that the ingredients can become bubbly and hot.

Sprinkle on the green onions and then serve right away.

Orange Chicken Supreme

Ingredients:

2 green peppers
2 ½ lbs. chicken thighs
2 Tbsp. oil
1 onion
Sauce
1 c. chicken broth
½ c. water
½ c. orange juice
2 tsp. orange zest
½ c. and 1 Tbsp. Splenda
¼ c. and 1 Tbsp. soy sauce
½ tsp. molasses
1/8 tsp. ginger
4 garlic cloves
1 tsp. sambal oelek
Thickener
½ tsp. xanthan gum

Directions:

To start this recipe, you can take the chicken and place it into a sealable bag. Take all of the sauce ingredients before pouring ¾ of a cup on the chicken. Seal up the bag and then let the chicken marinate for about an hour.

After the hour, drain out the chicken, making sure to save the marinade.

Heat up some oil in a wok before sautéing the vegetables so they become tender-crisp. Set the vegetables to the side before adding in the chicken and letting it cook so that there is no longer any pink left.

Add in the reserved and the leftover marinade and allow the chicken to simmer for another 15 minutes. Add in the xanthan gum to thicken the sauce.

Put the vegetables back into the wok and let them heat through before serving.

Meatloaf

Ingredients:

2 eggs
4 oz. cheddar cheese
1/3 c. ketchup
2 lbs. ground beef
2 garlic cloves
1 Tbsp. chili powder
1 Tbsp. Worcestershire sauce
1 tsp. cilantro
½ tsp. pepper
1 tsp. salt
Topping
¼ tsp. molasses
¼ c. ketchup
1 ½ tsp. Splenda

Directions:

To begin this recipe, turn on the oven and let it heat up to 375 degrees. Take out a bowl and mix together all of the meatloaf ingredients until they are well combined. In another bowl you will want to mix together all of the topping ingredients.

Place the meatloaf into a pan and brush on the topping. Place the pan into the oven and let it bake for an hour.

Serve this meatloaf right away and enjoy.

Philly Skillet Dinner

Ingredients

1 onion
1 lb. ground beef
8 oz. mushrooms
1 red pepper
1 green pepper
Salt
Pepper
1 garlic clove
4 oz. cheese

Directions:

Bring out a skillet and brown up the meat along with the onion until the meat is completely cooked through.

Add the garlic, green pepper, red pepper and mushrooms in next and let them stir fry so that the vegetables become tender and crisp.

Season this with the pepper, salt, and garlic clove before adding in the cheese. Cook until cheese is melted and then enjoy.

Dessert

Chocolate Nut Bars

Ingredients:

2 Tbsp. butter
1 oz. chocolate
2 Tbsp. cream
4 Tbsp. granular Splenda
2 Tbsp. syrup, sugar free
4 oz. almonds
1 c. chocolate protein powder
½ c. coconut, unsweetened

Directions:

Bring out a bowl and place the butter and the chocolate inside. Place these into the microwave and let them melt together for around a minute. Stir together until well blended and smooth.

At this time, add in the Splenda, syrup, and cream and blend well before adding the coconut, nuts, and protein powder.

Take out a baking pan and line it with some foil. Press this mixture into the bottom of the pan, making sure that it is even.

Place the pan into the refrigerator and let it chill until firm, which will take a minimum of two hours. Enjoy when done!

Peanut Butter Cups

Ingredients:

2/3 c. chocolate chips
½ tsp. butter
1 Tbsp. and 1 ½ tsp. peanut butter.
1 Tbsp. Splenda
12 peanut halves
1/8 tsp. vanilla

Directions:

Take all of the ingredients and place them into a bowl. Place the bowl into the microwave and melt everything together until it becomes smooth and well blended.

Pour this mixture into some candy cups and then put into the refrigerator in order to chill and set before enjoying.

Licorice Gummies

Ingredients:

¾ c. Splenda
½ c. water, cold
2 tsp. anise extract
2 pkgs. Gelatin, unflavored
1 drop food coloring, red

Directions:

Bring out a baking dish and mix together the food coloring, extract, Splenda, and water until well combined. Sprinkle the gelatin all over the water before stirring to combine.

Next, place the baking dish into the microwave and let it heat up for two minutes, stopping after a minute to stir well.

Pour this mixture into some loaf pans that are lined with some foil. Allow to chill for at least an hour so it can set.

When the gelatin has set, take it out of the pan and cut each of the bars into 8 pieces. Store until ready to use.

Puppy Chow

Ingredients

¼ c. chocolate chips
4 c. pork rinds
1 Tbsp. butter
2 Tbsp. peanut butter
¼ c. granular Splenda
1/8 tsp. vanilla

Directions

Begin this recipe by chopping up the pork rinds and placing into a bowl. In another bowl, place the butter, peanut butter, and chocolate chips and then let them melt together for about a minute, stirring in the middle. Add in the vanilla next.

Drizzle your chocolate mixture on top of the pork rinds, making sure to get them covered as best as you can. Spread out the pork rinds on a baking sheet and dust with the Splenda on both sides.

Place the baking sheet into the refrigerator and let it chill so the chocolate can set all of the way. Store or enjoy right away.

No Bake Cookies

Ingredients:

1 Tbsp. butter
2 tsp. cocoa
3 Tbsp. cream
2/3 c. sugar
2 Tbsp. oats
1 Tbsp. peanut butter
¼ c. almond flour
¼ c. coconut, unsweetened
¼ tsp. vanilla

Directions:

To start this recipe, take the cocoa, cream, Splenda, and butter and place into a saucepan. Allow the mixture to boil for about a minute, making sure to stir the whole time.

After this time, add in your peanut butter and let it stir so it is all well combined before adding in the rest of the ingredients.

Drop this mixture onto some wax paper and shape using your fingers. Place the wax paper into the freezer and let them become firm before enjoying.

Conclusion

Thank you for purchasing this book!

I hope this book helps you jumpstart your fat loss journey. If you enjoyed this book, then I'd like to ask you for a favor, would you be kind enough to leave a review for this book on Amazon.com. It'd be greatly appreciated!

Thank you and good luck!

Henry Brooke